Bob Merckel

SALUTE

for anyone who feels like
they're starting over

on or off the mat

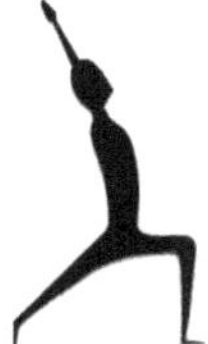

Contents

SALUTE

MOUNTAIN POSE
TADASANA

YOU ARE STANDING in *tadasana*, the mountain pose.

Your feet are planted firmly at the top of the yoga mat you keep at home. If you look out to the side, you can see the Mediterranean beckoning through the morning haze, but you look ahead. A pop-art Buddha you got in Siem Reap reminds you to focus.

You make sure you're in the proper position. Feet parallel, big toes touching at the top of the mat. You fan your toes to the best of your ability, which has never been all that great. Engage the thighs and think about rotating them slightly inward. Everything lifts up. Core is engaged. Shrug the shoulders and let them fall down and back. A quick tilt of the pelvis towards the legs makes sure all is correctly aligned.

You take a slow, deep breath and are ready to begin the first movement of Sun Salute A, aka *surya namaskara A*.

You pause.

It's been a while since you've done this. It's not like you don't know how. It's not like you haven't done literally hundreds, if not thousands, of these in the last 30-ish years. It's not like you didn't do around 40 of them a week for a few months when you started Ashtanga. Then you tore your adductor. A torn adductor does not a happy *asana* make.

You've been thinking about restarting your practice for several weeks now. You know you're better, but also keenly aware that does not mean fully recovered. Like your groin, your mind is torn between knowing the yoga could help to heal faster, but could also re-aggravate the injury. Perhaps you've been erring on the side of caution—petrified of pulling something new, or fucking up an injury that hasn't quite healed, or just being in pain.

There's been too much pain lately. You're not used to it, nor do you wish to be.

On the other hand, you don't want to be like all too many of the people you know, many of whom you love, who have lost their mobility.

These are the things you think about now, in your late-50s. How did that happen?

Your physio has assured you that you're good with forward movement. You are not so confident (and not yet cleared by the physio) with anything aggressive on the lateral front. But how much damage could a Sun Salute do? It's a warmup, basically.

It's a beginning.

You're standing at the beginning. You breathe in, thinking about the first movement, and exhale. You breathe in again.

You hate beginnings.

Hate is a strong word, so that's not exactly true. Beginnings make you anxious.

What you ~~hate~~ strongly dislike is starting over. It makes you feel like a failure—that you should never have stopped whatever you were doing, especially when it seemed you were making progress. Or felt like you were stagnating. You do this with running (which you've just been able to get back to, all so slowly). You do it with writing. You do it with keeping a gratitude journal. You do it with almost anything you say you're going to make a habit of.

Maybe your habit is starting over. Or more appropriately, putting off starting over until there is some internal or external catalyst that goes *kabang* and pushes you out of you comfort zone and back onto the starting block.

Maybe you need to be better about defining what you're embarking on and whether or not it actually means "starting over."

Maybe you need to just start and quit thinking about it.

You are standing tall. Go on, look at you! You *are* that fucking mountain.

Mount Tadasana, how noble you rise!

You breathe in, prepared for the first movement.

UPWARD SALUTE

URDHVA HASTASANA

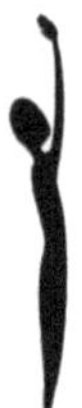

YOU'RE BACK ON the mat, centered and ready to begin. Feet firmly planted, outsides parallel and calloused big toes touching.

Looking down to double check, you resist the urge to pack it all in and head straight for a pedicure. Or maybe saunter up Calle Marina to All You Eat Is Love, the café you were in the other day that had a sign saying:

In this house
we do real
we do mistakes
we do I'm sorry
we do fun
we do hugs
we do second chances
we do happy
we do forgiveness
we do really loud

You bring your hands to prayer position in front of your chest. You breathe in and raise your arms above your head. You reach. Upward Salute. *Urdhva hastasana.*

The first real movement of Sun Salute.

You create a gentle tension in your body, feet still

pushing into the floor, grounding yourself. Your hands are reaching towards the ceiling, towards the sun.

It's a formalized version of one of the most basic stretches you do all the time. Grabbing something off the top shelf. Yawning indulgently. Holding an overhead rail on the bus or subway train. Helping someone shove that too-big-for-the-overhead into the overhead. Hailing a taxi. Getting rid of that cobweb in the corner (not right now but definitely before company comes). Standing in front of your students, writing UK slang they don't teach in textbooks at the top of the whiteboard: squiffy, does your head in, the dog's bollocks.

In the here and now, it's a controlled, precise movement. You look up and back towards your hands, palms pressed together. You feel you. Your core is taut. You feel a stretch in your chest and your heart opens just a little more. Your shoulders slide down and back. Your legs are solid, supporting the pose.

In the Ashtanga studio, the *shala*, you would be like this for only one inhalation. But you're at home so *no hay prisa, tranquilo.*

There is no hurry.

You take the time to breathe into the pose. You feel a tightness in your right shoulder, so you lean into that and stretch a little from side to side.

In this house we do real.

You close your eyes and lean further back, wondering what it will be like to return to back bends. You lose your balance a little but quickly recover.

In this house we do mistakes.

You move your hips around a little in a circular movement. It's not part of the practice, but you've been doing this a lot before and after runs, and it feels nice.

In this house we do fun.

You think about how many times you've rushed through this in the past, and how much you're enjoying getting back into it as slowly as is necessary. You feel you're growing taller with every breath.

In this house we do second chances.

You're starting to wake up, and smile at the thought of returning to your practice.

In this house we do happy.

You think about how long you've been out of commission, of the many reasons that might have caused that and that truly don't matter anymore. Of all the projects started, of all the races not run, all the round tuits you never got around to. You tell yourself it's all okay.

In this house we do forgiveness.

You take one more deep breath, reach a little higher, and let it out with the loudest "ahhhhh" you can manage. Banger, the scardiest of scaredy cats, jumps off the windowsill where he'd been sleeping.

In this house we do really loud.

You know you're ready to dive into the next movement, but for now we focus on this. And you know that in the entire practice you will have plenty of time to wrap yourself around yourself. You know you will flow back into this flow, into this series of movements, connecting your body to your breath, embracing each moment. The strength will come back, as will the flexibility. The folds, the twists, the squeezing of one muscle to release tension in another. Holding on to yourself while simultaneously trying to let go of anything but the present moment, the breath that you are in.

In this house we do hugs.

STANDING FORWARD FOLD
UTTANASANA A

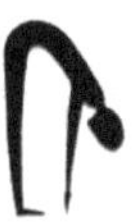

AS YOUR GYM teacher used to say, "touch your toes."

These days, especially on the first try, you touch your shins. And that is truly frustrating, because a few months ago, when you were in a regular practice, you could get down to your toes relatively easily. With legs straight! By the end of the warmup (five cycles of Sun Salutes), you could hang there with your knuckles pushing into the floor.

You have lost so much flexibility. You know it will all come back. But to what end? In about 12 hours you have a consult with a surgeon to see if or when an inguinal hernia needs to be repaired.

If that needs to happen sooner than later, then so be it. Get it done and get through the recovery and get back to it when it's safe.

If it needs to happen later, then it's probably better to be fit and flexible and all the more healthy for when they need to do the surgery. Doctor Google says recovery is only one to two weeks. Maybe you should talk to the actual medical professional before turning a "what if" situation into a worst-case scenario, but old habits die hard.

"It's not about the pose," your Ashtanga junkie friend has repeatedly said. "It's about the breath and the space."

In your heart, you know this is true.

That's a lie: you're not sure what the hell she's talking about. But you do believe you are where you are and in yoga, like in many other things, there is no perfect. There is no achieving one specific thing and then, *alakazam*, you're done.

You ponder how frustrating it is to get excited about something and join a few too many Instagram feeds only to see all these yogatastic Instamodels doing contortion poses.

You remember it is POINTLESS to compare. Yoga is not a competition.

You want to believe that.

You wish you believed that.

You know those reels are edited and photoshopped up the *asana* and back, that there have been dozens of outtakes before they posted just the right one. Even so, you still look at them and part of you goes, "well, fuck. I really wish I could do that / look like that. It will never happen. Why bother (re)starting?"

You also know the majority of them are 30 years younger than you are, and it's about the practice, not the unreasonably fit, semi-naked, fully flexible fitness models.

Moral of story: Instayogis do not make the best benchmarks.

What about the yogis in the Ashtanga studio? They are live. They are imperfect and they need adjustments. They don't always make it into the pose that is in the chart. But they are a million times closer to the ideal on the chart than you are.

Again. This is not a competition. They have been there longer than you, and surely they didn't start out as a fifty-something-year-old man recovering from a strained *gluteus medias* that kept him from walking without a limp for a few weeks (and that was before the torn groin. You are so falling apart.)

You are ridiculous.

The man you pay to help with your mental health wants you to reframe that thought. You overthink things, and that does not make you ridiculous.

Neurotic perhaps, but not ridiculous.

Just do the work. Breathe into where you are. Remember how much you improved from that first day in December until you had to stop at the end of February.

It is all a process.

Stand up.

Breathe in.

Reach to the sky.

Swan dive down, keeping your legs as straight as possible. Hinge at the hips and keep your back flat for as long as you can.

Your hands might only reach your knees. Your shins. The top of your feet. Maybe even your toes. It does not matter.

Move your weight to the front of your feet. You won't fall. Look, your fingers just got closer to the floor.

You only need to be there for that one exhalation. Relax your neck. Let your head fall down.

Release. Stay there for a few more breaths. Feel the stretch in your calves. Feel your hips release a little more.

Try to push up through your legs just a little bit. They don't have to be perfectly straight today. They don't have to be perfectly straight ever.

Just for fun, come back up very slowly.

This time, bend at your knees and try to fold your chest down on top of them. Don't worry about what you look like.

Your hands are on the floor. You said you couldn't do

that just a little while ago. Now push up and straighten out your legs as much as you can. That's enough. Don't overdo.

No one is taking your photo.

This is just you.

This is not for Instagram.

One more time. Inhale up into Upward Salute. Exhale slowly and swan dive down into Standing Forward Fold. Breathe there. Just hang there and be where you are right now.

Connect the breath to the movement.

Inhale up.

Stretch.

Exhale down.

Fall.

Try again.

Fall again.

Fall better.

HALF STANDING FORWARD BEND
UTTANASANA B

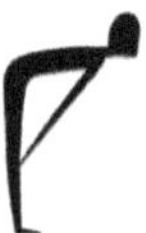

COMING UP OUT of *uttanasana A*, or Standing Forward Fold, you make the smallest of movements on the next inhalation. If there is any bend in your arms while folded over (and that's a big "if" for beginners), you push down and raise up into a flat back, while gently looking forward. But don't compress the back of your neck. It should be a smooth line from your hips to your crown; a nice flat back after having been folded over. This is *uttanasana B*, or Half Standing Forward Bend. This is the inhale before you jump back into *chaturanga*, which is when the real work begins.

In the yoga studios—Ashtanga Shala in Barcelona, Integral Yoga in New York, even at Ptown Gym—you loved this pose. It was a quick rest before the more strenuous bits; a relaxing inhale and stretch before getting down to business. It didn't matter if your hands didn't stay on the floor. When you go to flat back, your hands come up to your shins. Maybe a little lower when you're warmed up. Remember, this whole sequence you're exploring is done five times.

Sometimes you wonder why it's part of the sequence. Such a simple pose, not much of a change at all.

On a basic level, you know all the movements are connected to the breath. Inhale on upward movements, exhale when going down. The next movement is an explosive movement backwards, which requires an exhalation. So, you need to inhale after folding over and down on an exhale. Then, instead of simply inhaling in a static position, you keep the moving meditation going and rise up a bit on the inhale. This also puts us into a better position to jump back into *chaturanga*.

Maybe it's all about the flow.

Perhaps, it's like speaking different languages, where "rules" have developed to make the language flow more smoothly. For example, in English, you say "an" before a noun that starts with a vowel. Because it's easier to say "an apple" than "a apple." "A umbrella" sounds staccato, and is more difficult to pronounce. "An umbrella" flows.

You asked a friend who teaches and studies yoga if there was something more yogic or theoretical about going up into Half Standing Forward Bend. Were you missing something?

He said he thought of it in two ways. First, it prepares and trains the spine and core for jump backs, plank and *chaturanga*. But also, that 1-2-3 of folding over then extending the spine, to either fold again or jump back, increases mobility in the back, particularly the lower back.

Perhaps the yogis-that-be had something clever in mind when they decided on these compulsory sequences.

Maybe one day you'll be folded over so far you'll actually push yourself up into a flat back with hands on your mat. For now, it's just inhale, straighten your back as best you can, and look forward.

Not that *chaturanga* is anything to look forward to, but here you are.

FOUR-LIMBED STAFF POSE
CHATURANGA

YOU'RE ON YOUR mat.

The mat is on the beach, already a little sandy.

You've come to Somorrosto an easy five-minute walk from home, to salute the morning sun before it becomes blazing hot. You don't usually come here, tending to head left where there's a little more life—*chirringuitos*, volleyball matches, eye candy of all shapes and sizes. But today, early on a Sunday, Somorrosto seems almost soporific.

You've started the sequence and are in Half Standing Forward Bend, or flat back as you've taken to calling it. When you look up and out, you see a dozen or so yellow buoys of different shapes and sizes bobbing lazily on the calm Mediterranean. Further out are a pair of sail boats, and several cargo ships even farther. White wisps of clouds look airbrushed onto the Manganese blue sky.

A woman tentatively tries to balance on a paddleboard, her instructor talking her through it, already floating on the water.

You look back down and plant your hands into the mat, readying yourself to step back into *chaturanga*, the Four-Limbed Staff Pose that often makes you think of a train in Tennessee.

For you, it is the first bit of real exercise in the Sun Salute. So far, it's just been stretching a little; breathe in and look up, breathe out and fold down. You've been lulled into a false sense of security.

Suddenly you're self-conscious about exercising on the beach, about having brought your yoga mat, about debating whether to take your shirt off (you left the sunscreen at home, didn't you?) and thinking you should either go home or walk down another 20 minutes to your gym.

There are a few groups of people surrounding you, some of whom are sleeping in street clothes, others lying out in string bikinis and Speedos, and two guys behind you, drinking beers out of clear plastic cups, talking about their night at the clubs. They're speaking English in an accent you can't quite decipher.

You're sure that none of them are paying attention to you. Still, you can't help but feel that exercising amongst all these sand sleepers isn't going to be the right vibe.

The bespoke paddleboard class ebbs toward the horizon.

Everyone finds their balance in their own time.

You hear the guy behind you say, "the thing I love about Barcelona is that nobody judges you."

How had he gotten inside your head?

You're always self-conscious about getting into this pose. More seasoned yogis will jump back into a plank, then lower themselves down, elbows at their sides, until their entire body is like a board, parallel to the mat, supported by their feet and palms, elbows tucked into their sides at 90 degrees or less.

Those who have been practicing longer will seemingly float back into it rather than jumping. You believe this involves superhero levels of upper body strength, pelvic floor and core development, as well as hip flexor mobility—cards that you're just not holding right now.

It takes so much strength to appear graceful.

You suppose that's true off the yoga mat as well.

For now, you're back to basics, stepping one leg back at a time, slowly lowering yourself to as far as your arms will allow this morning. One step at a time. Focus on form. Focus on staying engaged. Don't worry about what you used to do, nor what you will be able to do. Just focus on the movement, as best you can do it, and the breath.

You decide to work on your core strength. Wanting to float one day is excellent motivation, and there's no need to rush through the sequence. You push back up into a straight-armed plank and breathe. You can hold these for at least a minute but rather than counting seconds (one Mediterranean, two Mediterranean), you count the sounds of the waves, rhythmically clapping into the shore. They're not so loud as to crash, more of a gentle woosh every few seconds.

Mother Nature's white noise.

You make it through five whooshes and decide to do two more planks.

Resting on your stomach, you feel the gentlest of breezes cooling the morning sun being. Your mat has absorbed quite a bit of heat.

Two older women, at least in their 70s, lay out their things in front of you, slowly stripping off *pareos* and sundresses, revealing string bikinis and skin as worn as your favorite jeans. They are tanned, wrinkled, saggy, and full of life, bantering quietly in Catalan. Either of them could be Mother Nature herself. They are gorgeous.

You push up back into plank after dusting some of the warm sand off your mat.

You count whooshes while a third elderly lady, sporting only the skimpiest of bikini bottoms, comes over from the left. They clearly all know each other, and the first two are complimenting the newcomer on her recent short buzz cut.

Six whooshes and you're done with the second plank.

As you recover, you see one of the guys who was sleeping has woken up and taken off his shirt. His back is a black and red medieval city, with a dragon flying above it. It's the one of the most amazing tattoos you've ever seen. In another life you'd go over and compliment him on it.

For now, you take in your surroundings, the recovering partiers, the sunbathers, the coven of sea goddesses in front of you, literally half-naked and so comfortable in their own weathered skins.

You feel foolish for having wondered about taking off your shirt. When did you become modest?

A plane slowly floats across the sky, headed to El Prat a few miles down the shore.

Tattoo boy's girlfriend blissfully sleeps while their other friend lights a joint.

A motorized boat, the size of a small fishing trawler, emerges from Port Olímpic to your left. It says *Escola Port* along its side. They train people how to navigate boats or even become yacht captains. You bet somebody on that boat could explain those yellow buoys.

You go into your third plank, thinking people are learning new things this morning: how to paddleboard, how to navigate a boat.

Two boys on paddleboards glide toward the shore. They are not novices. With practice comes grace.

You realize this applies to your yoga as well.

Three whooshes in and you lower yourself back into *chaturanga.*

The ladies are swimming.

The seagulls are squawking.

A corgi comes racing along the shore, nipping at the whooshes, its fur full of sand and its bark full of energy and joy.

You are on the mat, at the intersection of the city and the sea—a city that doesn't judge.

There's so much to see at sea level.

You are trying to be comfortable in your own skin.

The corgi barks again, reminding you to push into your next pose, Upward Dog.

UPWARD FACING DOG

URDHVA MUKHA SVANASANA

YOU TAKE YOUR mat to Ciutadella Park and wander around until you find a reasonably secluded spot. Away from the *manteros*. Away from the kids playing football. Away from the teenagers drinking *calimocho* (a local delicacy of cheap red wine mixed into a half-empty, 2-litre bottle of Coca Cola) and sway-bopping to their reggaeton. Away from the yapping terriers, play fighting for a stick. Away from the families pushing babies (and kids too old to be) in strollers.

You wonder as you wander, for the millionth time in your adult life, how peaceful it must be to feel so at ease that you can sleep anywhere in public, secure in the knowledge that mom or dad is there to push you around.

You pass an elderly lady in a wheelchair, also moving forward at someone else's behest. She seems to be awake, but just barely. You wish the Jamaican lady who is powering the wheelchair would stop just for a second, to wipe the speck of spittle off of the old woman's chin.

You find a tree to crawl under, it's almost like a canopy. Someone told you once it was a Japanese spindle tree. You have no reason to doubt them, but no real reason to believe. The Borrowers would find it enormous. You feel like Gulliver in Lilliput. You're painfully aware of mixing your literary metaphors, but that's the way your brain works today.

There you are. Sitting under a tree. Hello, Buddha.

Across the path, a girl is sitting near a hedge that seems to have purple foxgloves growing out of it. She's reading a paperback and you wonder if you shouldn't have taken your allergy medicine.

You arrange the mat so you'll be able to stand at the top, just outside of the canopy, but still in the shade.

You get up and center yourself. Take a deep breath in, come into *tadasana* for a few breaths. Birds are chirping. Locals are chatting indistinctly. Children keep going where their parents tell them not to.

You breathe in, raise your arms above your head, and look up towards your hands, placed together in prayer position. Your back bends backwards ever so slightly, and you feel the tiniest of pops.

Swing music, the gentle jazzy kind, is playing several hundred meters away. Barcelona is a dancing town and there are usually people in the big gazebo to your right, not too far from here, coming together to get their dance on. You remember that gazebo in Spanish is *glorieta*, which is such a lovely word. You also remember that this particular structure is called *Glorieta de la Transexual Sonia*, in memory of a trans woman who was murdered there in the early 90s by a group of neo-Nazis. The opposite of lovely.

So much joy, every weekend, in a place where something so horrific occurred not all that long ago. You think, "*Dios mío*, what a fucking world," and you shake it off and breathe in again.

The swing music is so happy. You try to come back after being sidetracked by Sonia. You realize you've never practiced to this kind of music, and it's a refreshing change.

You slowly breathe out into Standing Forward Fold and let yourself hang there for a couple of breaths. You remind yourself to drop your head instead of looking a little forward. Your hamstrings are so tight. The outside of your right knee asks if you truly want to do this today. It's hard to straighten your legs. Harder than usual. Everything will open up in time. Every day is different.

Breathe in, flatten your back, look forward. You see a folded piece of paper in your peripheral vision to your right. It says "task" and you wonder whose it was, whether they did it or not, and whether you should go have a look at it instead stepping back into *chaturanga*.

No. Your task is to get to the next pose in this sequence.

You inhale and try to jump back, because you're feeling sassy this morning and you had a good walk to the park so you feel a little warmed up despite your complaining thighs and knee.

It is not a graceful jump.

Lowering yourself down into Four-Limbed Staff you feel the back of your left shoulder pinch, just behind the scapula. There's a knot in there that you often tell massage therapists has been surgically implanted just to make their lives more challenging. Mental note: make a date to get on Kristo's table and have him hurt you in a good way.

Stay down here for a couple of breaths. The ground beneath the mat is softer than normal. More uneven. You note the irony of literally being on the ground yet feeling less grounded.

You can smell the dirt. The grass smells discernibly different than when it has been freshly cut. There's a woodsy aroma of twigs and fallen leaves coming in over the rubbery scent of your mat. It smells fertile, like something you could plant yourself into and grow.

A breeze blows in from your left, so refreshing.

Someone downwind is smoking weed.

From *chaturanga*, you exhale up into *urdhva mukha svanasana*, more commonly (and easily) called Upward Facing Dog. It's one of your favorite stretches. Odd how you think of this one as more of a stretch than a pose.

You push into the mat and straighten your arms. In theory, they become two pillars directly below your shoulders. While you're pushing up, you move your body forward ever so slightly, so that your feet roll over. In *chaturanga*, your weight is on your toes. In Upward Dog, your weight is on the tops of your feet.

It's strange how this happens. You haven't really thought about it all that much. You don't know how to describe it.

So you roll over and stretch your leg out in front of you, your foot facing up to the blue sky, perpendicular to your mat. You push your toes forward, as if you wanted to curl them down. They won't go all the way down, but the'll go forward and you can extend your ankle. It's actually quite simple. You're pointing your toes.

You flip back over and push yourself up into *chaturanga*. You straighten your arms and move slightly forward, pointing your toes as they roll behind you. Your right big toenail catches on the mat as this happens. You wince a little and decide maybe it is time for that pedicure.

Back into Upward Dog. Your weight's now on your palms and the top of your feet. Your legs are off the ground, your chest is high and open, your neck is long and your back is gently arched. In the studio you would do this all in one inhalation and breathe back into Downward Dog.

Since you're not in the studio, and you're getting into how this stretch really works, you exhale back into *chaturanga* and realize that's not as easy as you think and end up pushing yourself back into Child's Pose, which allows you to rest and think about how you go from having the tops of your feet on the mat to being propped up on your toes.

You realize that, while in your plank, you're not really going on the tips of your toes, but the bottoms of them, which are in effect grabbing the mat while the back of the feet push away at the joints where the toes meet the feet.

You think about the equivalent movement with your fingers vs your hands, and reckon the only time you would do this is when you're stretching to relieve/reduce carpal tunnel symptoms.

The girl across the path who was reading is now doing a shoulder stand next to her backpack. She didn't even bring a mat. Just lying there, the back of her shoulders and head on the ground her hands supporting her lower back, legs stretching up towards the sky. You hope she doesn't fall into the foxgloves.

You haven't done that inversion for years. It was a staple in the Hatha class you used to take in the West Village. They'd have you in it at the end of the practice for 2-3 minutes. It seemed like forever. It is in fact part of Ashtanga primary sequence, but much further down the road than you ever got.

You tell yourself to focus.

Back into *chaturanga*. Back into Upward Dog.

The strength of your arms pushing up drags the feet over and forward. Yes, that toenail needs to be clipped. Your spine lengthens forward and up. Although your lower back is bending, it doesn't feel compressed—always lengthening.

The shoulders and chest are broad and open. Keep lengthening by leading with your heart, not your head—it keeps your neck from pinching. Gaze down your nose.

Stretch from the front rather than thinking about

bending your back. If the breeze were coming from behind you, it would feel like your torso is a sail, billowing from the gentle pressure of the wind.

You stay here and enjoy the stretch, wondering how long you can keep your legs off the ground. It's okay to surrender, this is not easy to hold.

One breath in, one breath out.

You notice a statue in front of you, watching you practice. You will later learn that it's a monument to Marian Aguiló, a Spanish poet and linguist you had never heard of before. In the *shala*, there is a portrait of K. Pattabhi Jois, the founder of Ashtanga, whom you had never heard of until you started to practice. In Bikram, it was just Marc in his mesh dance shirt, yelling at you to stay on your mat.

Another inhalation. Your legs start to wobble so you let yourself play with your knees touching the mat and then coming back up.

A Pakistani man walks by holding a plastic shopping bag of cans. "*Cerveza*? *Agua*? Cold beer?"

You shake your head no, rather than saying, "are you crazy? I'm working here."

You can still hear the music coming from *Glorieta de la Transexual Sonia*.

You think you can make it a couple more breaths. A guy who has been lying on his stomach, just next to the statue of Señor Aguiló, rolls over onto his back and settles into a rather comfortable-looking position with his knees up and legs wide open. His shorts billow open in the breeze.

You wouldn't mind swing dancing with him.

You realize you are once again distracted and come back to the breath, to the stretch of your own torso. You take one more inhalation and raise your knees back off of the mat, preparing to push back into Downward Dog.

DOWNWARD FACING DOG
DHO MUKHA SUANASANA

WHAT IS DRIVING you to do this? Why the need to start over in this practice? Why the desire to start running again? What made you start in the first place?

What drives you to get off of the couch, or out of bed, and get back on your mat? To lace up those Sauconys?

You think it might be easier to just plant your heels into the mat than to explore these questions.

You're afraid of losing your mobility. You don't want to fall into the all-too-easy trap of "unfitness" that exists within the Venn diagram intersections of the people in your life. Your mom who couldn't walk across the living room without losing her stability. Your friend who couldn't ride a bicycle up a short hill last summer without thinking she was going to need an EMT. The pensioners on a cruise ship who couldn't move from buffet to buffet without their wheelchairs.

You were never an athlete. But at some point in your 20s you took Feldenkrais classes. Laurie called that movement for broken people.

You don't want to become one of the broken people. Yet here you are, 30 years later, recovering from a torn groin and waiting on a hernia surgery. This past year, you've felt closer to broken than you ever thought possible. Is this just a natural part of getting older?

You check your posture. Is your back rolling or are you keeping it flat? Twist those jars open, which helps to broaden your shoulders. Those with more flexibility run the risk of arching the spine. There will be no back bending here.

If you were in a studio, your instructor might push back and up on your hips, just a bit. Just enough to remind you to extend up and back, keeping your back flat.

You remember a yoga class at YogaNu on Greek Street in London. Could it have been a Downward Dog workshop? Yes, the instructor, Richard, was the one who taught you the "twisting of the jar lids" image.

He had you working in pairs. One person would be in Downward Dog and the partner would stand behind them. They would place a yoga strap across the front of your pelvis, and then take each end of the strap in their hands behind you. As you pushed into the mat, your partner would gently pull your hips back and up. Richard would come up alongside, place his palm on the small of your back, counteracting the pressure of belt. Suddenly your back felt lighter, as if there was a possibility to someday find rest in this pose.

Then you'd try to repeat that feeling without the strap.

When you were holding the strap, you got to see how it helped to subtly extend your partner's back. To create that flat line up from the mat.

The longer your back got, the easier it was to (almost) straighten your legs.

You breathe, trying to lengthen your back.

You remember the guy who ended up next to you in several of your Ashtanga sessions. He was a big fan of *Ujjayi* breath.

He made you self-conscious. You couldn't help but notice him. Were you not breathing loudly enough? Was he cos-playing Darth Vader? Were you doing something the wrong way?

Is yoga the right activity for a recovering perfectionist?

You breathe into the pose — not too loudly— conscious of your back, relaxing your shoulders, straightening your legs just a little more. No pain, just an uncomfortable awareness that you're pushing yourself a bit.

You think about going back to class. There are lots of videos and audios you can follow along with, but there is nothing like getting a little adjustment to help improve your practice. Not necessarily to do it perfectly, but to do it better.

It's all about doing it better. About being aware of where you are and realizing that, sometimes, you are improving. You are not starting over. You are starting again with experience.

You breathe in one last time here, in this sequence within the sequence, a little more aware of some of the experiences that have driven you to this breath. And you're very aware that there are many more to reflect upon when you have more time.

But for now, you prepare to step forward, back into *uttanasana B.*

HALF STANDING FORWARD BEND (AGAIN)

UTTANASANA B

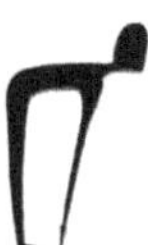

YOU'VE TAKEN TODAY'S practice to the pier across the street from your house. It overlooks Bogatell beach, which is too packed with volleyball players to find space to unroll the mat.

There's so much going on, it's almost distracting. You're once again only five minutes away from your quiet apartment, this time you turned right. Amazing how one can cross the street and end up in another universe.

You breathe in, straighten your back, and look up.

A volleyball shoots up directly beyond the wall. Higher than any game would call for. You can see one row of volleyball courts, and you know there is another row directly on the other side of the wall. Somebody in the hidden courts must be showing off. The ball rockets up; a good 30 meters in the air. No parabolic curve. You half expect it to pop open and have an army of toy soldiers burst out, with plastic parachutes opening, all of them gliding to safety.

You breathe in, straighten your back, and look up.

A couple of miles ahead looms the huge solar panel structure, the *photovaltaic*, in Parc del Forum. Last week you were in that park, weaving your way through throngs of festival-goers, on your way to see Carly Rae Jepson (the newly crowned queen of underground pop). Then Miley Cyrus (who earned a new level of respect, you hadn't realized she could truly sing), Janelle Monáe (worth twice the price of admission), and finally Robyn (who had the masses singing and crying at the same time). This year's Primavera Sound should've been rebranded Prideavera. It was poptastic; another different universe, just a 25-minute walk away.

You breathe in, straighten your back, and look up.

A DJ inside the nearby restaurant window plays chillout music that gently trip hops into your head. A party of Colombians sits around the terrace table directly below him, the guest of honor with baby's breath in her hair. They seem a little dressed up for a day at the beach.

They have one little boy with them. He's dressed in a blue seersucker suit (short pants), and light blue matching sneakers. He keeps running over to the wall with a toy firetruck in hand (another volley rocket shoots up). Sometimes he races it along the benches, sometimes he stands there, looking out over the beach like Simba on Pride Rock. It's a good 15 meters down. He teeters too close to the edge—clearly not in mountain pose—looking over and glancing back towards his mother. He has the most beguiling of impish grins. One that clearly lets him get away with anything. One gust of wind and he'd be gone, with no toy soldier parachute.

You want to tell his mom to put down her *cerveza* and look after her boy, but that's not your battle.

You breathe in, straighten your back, and look up.

A few days ago, it was too chilly to dip your toes. Now, it's the beginning of tourist soup. Paddleboarding students glide across the swells, reminding you to learn to do that one season. It was supposed to happen two summers ago, but you opted for padel lessons instead—the court sport, not standing on oversized surfboards and propelling yourself with oars.

"That waterboarding looks fun," Doug said one afternoon.

You were sitting at Vai Moana, this year's *chirringuito* of choice just up Bogatell, sharing a bottle of overpriced Rioja (you pay for the view) and *patatas bravas*.

He pointed to three paddleboarders just past the buoys, one noticeably wobblier than his friends.

"Waterboarding is very, *very* different," you said. "Google it."

Down along the beach where you'd run the other day, they offer paddleboard yoga. As if balancing on one leg and bending forward isn't challenging enough, why not try it while floating on a moveable surface?

You breathe in, straighten your back, and look up.

Two women in hippie dresses have taken a seat on Pride Rock, directly in your line of sight. Beaded purses, feather earrings. One smoking a fag and swirling around what looks like a white plastic bottle of liquid yogurt. They haven't put on enough sunscreen and their shoulders will be having words with them tonight in their hotel beds.

You breathe in, straighten your back, and look up.

The people standing on the beach are casting shadows twice as long as themselves. The volleyball players show no intention of winding down and you wonder where they get all the energy. The kid with the fire truck has been temporarily distracted with *churros con chocolate*, and that seersucker will never come clean. The lady with the feather earring has the longest yawn you've ever seen. It is contagious. It's time to cross the street. To return to the quiet universe of home, where a gentle stretch awaits you before dinner.

STANDING FORWARD FOLD
(AGAIN)

UTTANASANA A

YOU ARE ALMOST back to the beginning. You're a little more warmed up than you were the first time you were here. You're also definitely a little more out of breath. You can feel the perspiration starting to form on the back of your neck and forehead. Once you finish, you've got four more of these Sun Salutes ahead.

Your fingers touch the mat much more easily this time. You're still a long way from having your palms on the floor. That said, you realize those five breaths in Downward Dog are starting to do their trick. Your legs feel looser. Maybe even stronger, a bit more engaged. You notice a drop or two of sweat on the mat that wasn't there when you unrolled it a little while ago. You know by the end of the sequence you'll feel more comfortable, and you'll see more sweat. Your MacBook in the other room notifies you of a message.

You focus on the stretch in your hamstrings and try to hinge from your hips. Lean a little forward, weight in the toes as they push into mat — it will help you straighten your legs. Relax your …

That Facebook group you'd been chatting in before your practice is going into DefCon four. You really should have closed the laptop before you started to practice. You wonder what everyone is so chatty about, but you also know it will not be earth shattering.

You focus on your balance. On folding over and hanging there, taking a few extra breaths. Your legs look too white for the beginning of shorts season. You'll have to start over on your tan as well.

You remember the boss you had in New York, the Parisian executive who lived in Brussels and would ring you up to ask you if you had received his emails, and if so why hadn't you responded. You couldn't very well say, "I was doing a Sun Salute, J.B." But you could tell him you'd been in a meeting or finalizing his presentation or in the middle of composing a response to his email. It didn't matter. Nothing was ever quick enough for him.

You breathe back into Half Standing Forward Bend, not so much that you want to go backwards, but because you want to focus on folding into *uttanasana*. You feel your heels come back into the gentle cushion of the mat.

You really need to change the sound of that notification. Or turn it off. You remember being on a train one morning, heading home from a late night out in Tarragona. You were supposed to have been home the night before, but sometimes you have to go with the flow. You had bought a business ticket in the "quiet car"—not because you're fancy, but because you craved silence and the possibility of catching up on an hour's sleep.

The man across the aisle was talking on his phone. He had another on the tray in front of him, constantly vibrating and going "choo choo." Whoever told him that a train whistle Whatsapp notification would be cute was wrong. You also remember that when he did stop talking, and started responding to his texts, that he had never turned off the keyboard "click" sound. Click click click.

Choo choo. *"Dime... vale vale... estoy en tren."*

It. Was. The. Quiet. Car.

You say nothing because a) you avoid confrontation, especially in a second language, and b) you like to think of these things as Buddhist challenges. Breathe through them and let them just pass. Sure, the story is in the confrontation, but better to sit in self-righteous indignation than get flustered trying to tell the man to have some respect for other people's personal space. Nothing last forever. You'd lived through two years of JB, you can make it through an hour-long train journey.

You breathe in and out, hanging here in the fold, feeling yourself let go. You try to disconnect from your thoughts. You try to disconnect from the dinging Facebook page. You focus on the present. Breathe into your hips and see if they can't release some more. You notice a scratch on your shin that you have no idea where it came from. You see little tears on your mat, where the cat has decided it makes an excellent scratching pad.

You connect to the breath and try not to pay attention to the dings and scratches. You wonder why it is so hard for people to disconnect these days. Why people need to have personal phone conversations right next to you on public transport. Why people, especially here in Spain, were never taught the concept of inside voices.

You breathe one more time and sink a little further down; connected to your breath and, trying not to judge yourself or others, still connected to the distractions of your own devices as well as those on the coffee table in the other room.

You think about your eventual return to the *shala*. The mat there has no scratches. It's had no life outside of the studio. There is another benefit to practicing there. There are no technological distractions in the studio. You don't stop in the middle to answer a WhatsApp. You do the work. You don't stop in the middle to adjust your notifications. You do the work. You don't stop in the middle to add your two cents to the latest "can you believe what she posted?" in the Facebook group.

You breathe. You release. You do the work.

You think about your home practice. About the distractions.

You wonder if you could leave them, say goodbye. Left to your own devices, you probably would not.

You breathe.

Later, when you get to the Facebook group, you find out the fitness app you all belong to had fired even more people, and the running coach you all had taken against had posted even more beige food on her Insta.

Better that you stayed with the practice.

UPWARD SALUTE (AGAIN)
URDHVA HASTASANA

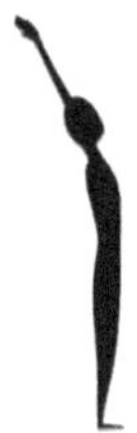

IT'S TIME TO move forward again. To push yourself back up towards the mountain.

Back to the start. Doing the same thing over and over. Is there power in this repetition or is it self-inflicted punishment? Sisyphus did the same thing over and over—a punishment for having tricked the gods.

While sometimes this practice may seem punishing, you don't see it as a punishment. You are on an adventure where, by focusing on the present, you might end up at the same place, but you will have spent time becoming more aware of yourself, and perhaps made progress along the way. Some trips up this hill are easier than others. Sometimes the boulder rolls more smoothly, other times you feel it's weight might roll back and crush you.

But you are no masochistic Sisyphus. You are here because you're committed to the process. To becoming more aware of the breath and the space. Plus, you know you will feel better for having faced today's challenges.

As you inhale, you rise back up into Upward Salute. You realize you've been here before. The poster on the bookshelf in your office-cum-home-studio reminds you:

This Must Be the Place.

You are where you are, and this is where you're meant to be. Your lower back bends backwards with a touch more freedom. The backs of your legs feel straighter and don't seem as tight. Your hips feel more open.

You prepare to repeat the raise, because you can.

Before you bend down and then reach to the sky, like that beach volleyball shooting straight up a few days ago, you take some time to reflect. Who else do you know who's ended up, at least physically, just where they started?

The circular narrative, that's what they call it.

Dorothy ended up back in Kansas. Alice woke up on the riverbank after falling down the rabbit hole.

One could argue that Dorothy did not choose to go to Oz, but once she arrived, she was determined to get back home. She did what she was told, went through all number of adventures (isn't each *asana* an adventure?) in order to complete her cycle. Do you need brains, a heart, and courage to practice yoga?

Wisdom comes from the practice. You learn more about your body, and your resolve, each time you practice.

If you don't have a heart, or compassion, especially for yourself, you probably won't enjoy your practice. It will just be pushing that boulder up the mountain every time you get to the mat. With compassion comes the patience you need to accept where you are. Some days are better than others; today (or this week, or this month) you won't be able to do what the yogi on the mat next to you is doing. But maybe next week, next month, you'll do what you're doing now a little better. A little deeper. A little smoother.

You need courage to try new things, to believe you're not going to fall when you fold forward, to trust that your back will bend a little more when the teacher presses down on you.

To get back on the mat after pulling your adductor.

To get back on the mat and stay there.

It takes courage to start again. It takes courage to admit you're afraid and do it anyway.

In Siem Reap last January, you started talking to the couple next to you eating Cambodian barbecue. Two Colombians who had been living in the German-speaking part of Switzerland for the past 15 years. They were in Siem Reap for a few days before heading to a Cambodian beach for a 7-day Ashtanga retreat. They fell down the Ashtanga hole about eight years prior and most of their subsequent holidays were spent on yoga retreats.

Was it not a trifle surreal to be sitting on a sidewalk in Southeast Asia talking about something you'd only started thinking about a few weeks before? Laughing about how some postures seemed impossible to ever master, yet others had either been accomplished (not perfectly, never perfectly) or were on their way to feeling more comfortable.

Had you not fallen down your own rabbit hole of YouTube videos, yoga apps, and Instagrammers who offered guidance how to jump back; how to do a handstand (another Insta obsession); how to master Downward Dog (you will never be that dog's master, but you might teach it to stay)?

Sun Salute, and the entire Ashtanga practice in general, is showing up and doing the same thing over and over.

It is the Groundhog's Day of yoga. Are we Phil Connors every time we step onto the mat? Destined to repeat the same day until we find redemption?

Maybe not redemption, but you do know you gain a little more self-awareness each time you practice. Every time you step on the mat, you come with a little more knowledge, a little more compassion. You're aware of a different experience, even though it might seem familiar to the unobservant observer. And when you finish, you say job done—until the alarm blares and you start all over again the next morning.

What do you need to do to make this yogic loop a better experience?

Do you need companionship in Ashtanga? You rely on your teachers to help you grow. To nudge you into better form, to give you the next postures in the sequence. To hold you up when learning balancing poses, when you would otherwise fall.

You rely on your friends who also practice to let you know they've struggled too. To give you tips from the trenches. They have been there before you and teach you to be patient with yourself.

You rely on the others in the studio, even though you may never speak to them, because they are physical manifestations of what seems to be the impossible. Full lotus? Legs behind your head? Clasping your own hands behind your feet in a seated forward bend? These are circus tricks on the Internet, but in the *shala* they seem like accomplishable tasks.

You take another breath.

This round of Sun Salute is almost over.

And yet the journey is just beginning.

MOUNTAIN POSE (AGAIN)
TADASANA

YOU BORROW A mat from the hotel spa and walk across the street to the park on the other side of the promenade, the one where you'll run later on today. It's full of palms and cactii. There are cypress trees and one particularly giant rubber tree (or is it a fig?). You were never good with trees, but you like to do the pose.

You unroll the mat in a corner of Parque Genovés. It's not like Park Ciutadella in Barcelona. The gazebo here looks like a spaceship, much larger than the one back home. Nobody is swing dancing, but there's a dad playing tag with his three kids and they seem to be having fun. The mat is thicker than the one you've been using, more cushion on top of the springy ground; a different give, the texture somewhat stickier than the older, more worn-down one you use at home. But the mat feels strangely familiar even though it's new to you.

It's like kissing someone new — it usually feels sort of the same, but you never know quite what to expect and it takes a while to get comfortable with the differences.

You ease yourself through the Sun Salute sequence.

You are a mountain surrounded by trees. The breeze is cooler than you ever thought it would be this time of year in the south of Spain. You can hear the gurgle of fountains not far away. The air smells green.

You inhale into Upward Salute and exhale into Standing Forward Fold. It's your first one of the days, but you realize you can go further into it than when you restarted the practice a couple of months ago. And yet here you are, restarting.

Half Standing Forward Bend then push back into *chaturanga*, exhaling back into Downward Dog. The stretch feels so good after 8 hours of train travel yesterday. It's still not a resting pose (will it ever be?), but you feel well-rested and take five breaths while pedaling one heel after the other into the mat. You think about maybe taking a bike tour and pedaling around Cadiz. Then step forward, returning into Half Standing Forward Bend. Dad is taking his kids to the fountain. You'd noticed earlier his fading commitment to the game. You are in awe of the Dragon Tree on the other side of the gazebo. A giant monk of a tree, its thick branches forking into smaller ones, reaching up not out, covered by a tonsure of leaves.

You breathe out and fold over into *uttanasana*. It seems easier today than yesterday, maybe because you're doing it after a lot of walking last night, first through the labyrinth of town to see the Plaza de España: is there one in every Spanish city? And why does this one feel so *tranquilo* yet monumental? Then a stroll back through the *maravilla* that is the Alomeda Apodaca with its giant fairy-tale ficus trees, magnificently tiled fountains, and bougainvillea-laden trellises. Then to rest on an unexpectedly comfortable wrought-iron bench, soaking in the Atlantic breeze, trying to discern what differentiates it from the Mediterranean air you were breathing yesterday.

Your fingers splay out on the mat and you see the

tiniest of beetles has joined you in your practice. You watch how he suddenly stops as if he's realizing "hey, this isn't grass anymore, how'd that happen?" You picture him look around, shrugging his thorax and saying, "it is what it is" as he restarts his gentle journey to the other edge of the mat. You're so zen you're attracting the local fauna. Next it'll be those ducks by the fountain, waddling over for a visit.

You inhale up, back into Upward Salute. It's the last inhalation of this round of Sun Salute. And you're doing it under the Andalusian sun, bright and suspended in the clearest of blue skies in a public garden you'd only heard of last week.

You cannot help but squint. Despite the chilly sea breeze, the sun warms your upstretched neck. The mat feels squishy and solid beneath your feet.

Your legs are engaged and your back arches backwards more smoothly than the first breath of today's practice.

You breathe in again, grateful for the extra breath, for the extra moment in this posture.

You exhale, lowering your arms and placing them in prayer position. One Sun Salute complete. Surrounded by other yogis in a studio, you'd be doing five more of these.

But here in this park amongst the trees, you lift your right foot and place it as high up as you can against the opposite inner thigh.

You engage your left thigh muscles, pushing down into the squishy solidness. You focus on something that will not move. That V where a branch of the dragon tree forks out into two. Unmoved by the wind, you stand solid under his tonsure. You have your balance for now. You know it is fleeting and often takes a series of micro-adjustments to stay there. You wish you had something to hold onto as you start to lose the pose. You waver. You drop your leg. You breathe and go back into it. Your hip is still tight, but not like it was several months ago. You try to open up just a little more, to bring the knee back into a line parallel with your hipbones. Your *gluteus medias* says, "not that far." And you realize you are where you are and that's okay.

You are where you are.

You breathe.

You balance.

You are in a park surrounded by trees hundreds of years old in a city founded in 1104 BC.

You breathe into the pose. You breathe into the balance. You breathe into how short these breaths are, how old this ground is.

You slowly bring your foot down. You place it on this mat that isn't yours and center yourself.

You raise your left foot up, placing your heel into the top of your right inner thigh. There is no pain on this side, nor discomfort in your adductor as you slowly rotate it out. You are healing. You think it has taken forever, but it's just been a moment.

Your pain. Your discomfort. Your breath. Your distractions. They are just moments.

Engage the right thigh.

Ground the right foot into the mat.

You breathe.

You balance.

You take in this moment of peace. You take in the fact that yesterday you were so fraught with anxiety you almost cancelled the trip.

The fountains. The traffic. The ducks. The palms. The breeze.

You hear your breath, quiet.

You breathe.
You balance.
You lower your leg. The tree becomes the mountain.
You smile and realize you are crying.
You realize you might not be that balanced.
You are where you are.
You breathe.

THE RETURN

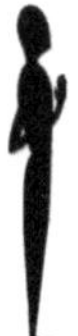

YOU'RE IN PROVINCETOWN. You don't have a mat.

You told yourself the other day that when you got to the Cape you would take a yoga class the next morning. Getting back to the Ashtanga studio was impossible in Barcelona, but a class here could be interesting. You woke up ridiculously early (hello, time zones) and tried, without much success, to make sense of the scribbling you did over the past few days. You've been feeling disjointed and your discourse reflects it. Doug wanders downstairs, still half asleep, and you tell him you're going to yoga class at 10 o'clock. He squints at his watch and says, "well, you've got an hour and a half," which seems like just enough time to find a second cup of coffee and some motivation.

Something seems a little off kilter and you think you'd better check that course time again. The gym's webpage tells you it starts at nine and you're like, well I guess that's yoga tomorrow then.

Ten minutes later, you're at Provincetown Gym paying for a week's membership and talking to a new girl named Phina, which you find out is not short for Philomina. Joey—who you've known for years around town, was

Doug's trainer last summer and now owns the place—waves from the middle of the gym and mouths "Hi, Bob" while counting out reps for his client. Like the TV song says, sometimes it's good to be where everybody knows your name. Even if it's been a year since your last visit.

You wait outside the exercise room for the kickboxing class to end. Rodrigo, the Brazilian fireman, is teaching it and he's hotter in person than in his pictures.

An Earth mother comes up to you and asks if you're there for the yoga class. Her hair is shorter than yours has ever been and she has one feather dangling from her right ear. She looks nothing like the woman on Pride Rock a few weeks ago. Her plastic rimmed glasses say I'm artsy but not pretentious. She looks like someone who would gladly give you a hug if you asked, and perhaps if you didn't, and you would feel immediately safe and warm.

You point to the mat rolled up under her arm, say it looks like she is, too. "I'm teaching it, actually."

Her name is Kate and you tell her it's your first class in months, you're recovering from a couple of injuries but you've been practicing on your own this month, and writing a bit about that. You don't know why you feel compelled to share that.

"Oh, great! I'm a writer, too. It's a very gentle class. Do what you can, don't do what doesn't feel right. Listen to your body. Listen to me as well, but to your body more. It's a journey of a thousand steps."

Rodrigo and his kickboxers leave the space and you head in with a few other women and one little man, who is older than you and looks very serious about his practice. They all have their own mats, which you do not. You grab one of the black rubber mats hanging over rail on the wall. It's light and spongy and doesn't look like it will be sticky at all. You take a space in the center and flop the mat down gracelessly.

Another older woman comes in, obviously a local, and tells the woman in front of me that she looks like her friend Barb. Not-Barb says, "No, I'm Linda but I look like everybody."

"I don't know that you look like everybody," says the newcomer with the South Boston accent, "but I'm telling ya, you look like Barb."

Meanwhile, Kate is catching up with the others who are settling onto their mats. Jennie, who seems like she's in her early 30s, is from Wyoming and hasn't done much since last week's class. Adriana is young and limber and lithe, the only one of us who looks like a dancer. The old guy up front isn't saying much. You think about the shift from kickboxing to yoga, and you settle onto your mat.

You tell yourself any room can be a yoga room and you remember a meme that said, "How do I get a yoga body? 1. Have a body. 2. Do yoga."

The class begins on the floor. The mat is mushy. Much more so than the one you borrowed in Cadiz. This feels more like something you'd put under a sleeping bag. You're on the ground floor and the door at the end of the room is open. It's a foggy morning and the room smells of damp and kickboxers. The mat smells faintly of plasticized rubber. It's been used, cleaned and re-used so many times that it has just taken on a banal aroma of "yes, I live in a gym, but I'm clean. How can I help you?"

You follow Kate's instructions. They are neither hurried nor especially demanding. She who looks like a giver of hugs is having you hug yourself, gently warming up your back and legs by kneading them with your hands. Simple stretches, bringing breath into the lungs, blood into muscles, movement into the joints.

You feel like you are warming up for a practice. You

wonder if this is the practice.

You end up in tabletop and do some balancing and stretching. Bird dog, you think it's called. It's core work that your physio has recommended.

Kate says, "'5 A.M. in the Pinewoods,' by Mary Oliver" and begins reciting a poem. You've never been in a yoga session slash poetry recital. You try to listen to the words as you focus on the breath and not straining your invisible hernia. Instead, you remember the surgeon saying, "It's not bad now, but we want to repair it before it gets worse. You'll know if that happens, and it will not be pleasant."

You've had several unpleasant dreams about that. You focus on the poem instead which is not about a dream.

You breathe and push your right hand into the mat. You bring your left elbow into your right knee. Your adductor whispers, "hello, I'm still here."

Kate gently recites more Oliver telling you this is how you flow outward, this is how you pray.

You go into plank from tabletop.

You see that Laura-not-Barb is now standing on her mat, leaning against the wall. You've never seen this particular modification and as we go down into a very floor-based *chaturanga*, you try to focus on your own floor work, at the same time fascinated by LnB's wall work.

You realize that, just like in Ashtanga, there are modifications for everyone. Even though you, who still feel like you are starting over, think this is a relaxing start to the practice, there are people who starting over from different places. And you have this surge of affection for this woman who is making this moment her own, working to the best of her capabilities.

Be kinder to yourself in your own practice. Find your own flow. Find your own way how to pray.

After a while, we all join Laura on our feet, and come

into a standing position at the top of our mats.

"We're going to do some Sun Salutes," Kate tells us.

You've been preparing all month for this.

You breathe in to Upward Salute. You move back because your hands hit the ceiling beam above you. You breathe out into Forward Fold. Your legs are warmed up and this feels gentle and familiar, like a forward fold after several sun salutes at Ashtanga.

Breathe in, flat back, look forward. You see two muscle boys in tank tops walking outside the open door, heading to the gym's entrance which is around the corner.

You exhale out to push back into...

No. This is not what Kate says.

She tells you to go back into Forward Fold, slightly bend the knees and flow back up into Upward Salute.

When is a Sun Salute not a Sun Salute?

You repeat this a few times while she recites another poem, "Labyrinth." You later wish you could remember the lines. The mazes you've been in, the puzzles you've had to solve to get here. The queues going through security and immigration, the winding cobblestone streets in Andalucía, Parc del Laberint d'Horta on the edge of Barcelona that you've been meaning to go to for years. The wrong turns you've made and the pretty houses you've seen as a result.

You go into various warrior poses. They are familiar and yet different. The mat stretches under your feet. It has a lot of give, but you feel it will rip like foam rubber. And then there goes your torn adductor again.

You continue with cautious awareness.

You do what feels right for your body. You're in Warrior Two. She tells you to lean forward into your future. Come up to your present. Lean back to your past, just for a breath. Come back to the center. Come back to the present.

You go back down to the floor. More planks. Side planks. You haven't tried those in a long time. They feel more comfortable than you would imagine.

You're getting better.

You follow Kate's voice. She leads you into child's pose. She says to stay there and relax into it. Breathe into where there is tightness. Breathe into your hips. The small of your back. Your knees which you feel are slowly relaxing. You wonder how close the others' butts are to their heels. You wonder if you will be able to sit on your heels again without pain. You don't look at the others even though you are curious.

Kate says to keep breathing and hold this position. While you're there, she will come around and give you each a short back massage, if you are comfortable with that. If not, place one palm up to the ceiling and you won't have to be touched.

You do not turn your palms.

She pulls your shirt back tight along your back. You immediately feel protected. She massages your right trapezoid and then the left, then both. She cups your shoulders in her hands. They are stronger than you had imagined. She pats you on the back as she finishes.

Good boy.

You are moved by her touch. By her strength. By her gentleness. By the words she recites. Another poem, this one's name you did not catch.

We roll over into *savasana*. We breathe into our corpses. We feel fiery balls of energy in our hands, their golden lava flowing up our arms, into our bodies, energizing us for the day ahead. We roll over on to our sides. She tells us to stay fetal for a few breaths. You are not used to being guided out of *savasana*.

From corpse pose into fetal position.

We are being reborn.

Starting over. Always starting over.

We come up into a seated position and do one final breathing sequence. We chant an ohm. We recognize the light in ourselves and we extend it to the others around us. We bring our hands in front of us, one final stretch, and *namaste*.

You see that Laura-not-Barb not only bows to her own light, but makes an effort to give a bow and a namaste to each of us in the room.

Your feel her light. It makes you smile with your whole being.

You'd felt part of a community coming into the gym, now even more so. Now your community is made up of people you have never met.

You look forward to your day. To the morning fog burning off. To seeing old friends. To going into town. To getting a new yoga mat. To bringing it to the gym tomorrow morning, when once more you will be back on the mat.

ACKNOWLEDGEMENTS

Thank you to all my teachers and instructors, but most of all to Shaun Levin. He's been with this project for more than five years; the literary yogi that has gently nudged me to stretch a handful of writing exercises into a fully formed book.

An abundance of gratitude to Michelle (who was there at the beginning) and the rest of Shaun's Creative Sundays group, without whom I might never have unrolled this mat. Valerie, Pia, Joyce, Joanna, Pawel, SJ, Cynthia, Zurina, Ann, Rachel, and Holly—y'all are the best.

To Larry, all my love and thanks.

BOB MERCKEL is a writer, editor and language teacher who spends his time between Barcelona and Provincetown. He holds an MA in Creative Writing (Novels) from City University London. His work appears in *Tales of the DeConstructed*, *Your Messages*, and Medium, amongst others. A recovering corporate marketing exec, he now happily teaches English at a Catalan university.

@bobzyeruncle

9 798329 005783